@**Copyright 2018by** Daisy M. Ortc

This document is geared towards providir information in regards to the topic and iss. is sold with the idea that the publisher is not required to render accounting, officially permitted, or otherwise, qualified services. If advice is necessary, legal or professional, a practiced individual in the profession should be ordered.

Under no circumstance will any legal responsibility or blame be held against the publisher for any reparation, damages, or monetary loss due to the information herein, either directly or indirectly.

Legal Notice: The book is copyright protected. This is only for personal use. You cannot amend, distribute, sell, use, quote or paraphrase any part or the content within this book without the consent of the author.

Disclaimer Notice: Please note the information contained within this document is for educational and entertainment purposes only. Every attempt has been made to provide accurate, up to date and reliable complete information. No warranties of any kind are expressed or implied. Readers acknowledge that the author is not engaging in the rendering of legal, financial, medical or professional advice. The content of this book has been derived from various sources. Please consult a licensed professional before attempting any techniques outlined in this book.

Table of Contents

What is Lectin?... 6

Why has eliminating lectin from your diet become important?.... 7

Foods containing Lectin.. 9

Choose the substitutes.. 11

Cooking and processing methods which help in reducing the quantity of lectin in diet... 13

Say no to these foods.. 15

Say yes to these foods... 16

Take away message.. 18

Introduction.. 19

Chapter 1 – Salad Recipes... 20

    Roasted Artichoke Salad.. 20

    Salmon Salad with Orange and Cheese............................. 22

    Sweet Potato Salad with Vegan Cilantro Pesto.................. 24

    Kale Salad with Ham.. 26

    Ham and Arugula Salad with Sweet Potato....................... 27

    Steak Salad with Yogurt Dressing...................................... 29

    Peaches and Berries Salad with Spicy Tahini Dressing..... 30

    Shrimp Salad with Herbed Vinaigrette.............................. 31

    Sweet Potato with Chipotle Salad and Tahini Dressing.... 33

Chapter 2 – Vegan Ice Cream Recipes.................................... 35

    Superfood Ice Cream with Cacao Nibs.............................. 35

Chocolatey Avocado Ice Cream.. 36

Cauli-Banana Ice Cream.. 37

Vegan Vanilla Ice Cream... 38

Strawberry Ice Cream... 39

Avocado and Raspberry Ice Cream Squares... 40

Chapter 3 – Breakfast Recipes... 42

Cheesy Breakfast Burritos... 42

Flourless Garlic Breadsticks... 44

Shirataki Fettuccine Pasta with Artichoke and Basil.............................. 46

Protein Energy Balls with Dried Blueberries... 48

Cauliflower Risotto with Mushrooms.. 49

Tasty Mushroom Soup..51

Baked Peach Cobbler Pancakes... 53

Cassava Flour Pancakes with Cinnamon... 55

Cream of Asparagus Soup... 57

Cauli Rice with Lime... 58

Chapter 4 – Main Course Recipes..59

Cheesy Chicken Enchiladas with Adobo Sauce....................................... 59

Yummy Salmon Cakes.. 61

Shirataki Angel Hair Pasta with Avocado Sauce..................................... 63

Chicken Strips with Cilantro Dipping Sauce... 64

Cauli Rice with Basil Pesto... 65

Veggie-Filled Fettuccine Alfredo..67

Baked Okra Bites... 69

Vegan Fudgy Tarts..71

Baked Sweet Potato Toast... 73

Walnut Fudge... 75

Tasty Gingerbread in a Mug..76

Ravioli with Basil Pesto... 77

Chapter 5 – Soup and Appetizer Recipes..79

Mint and Berry Soup... 79

Spiced Cauliflower Rice Soup... 81

Swiss Chard Fritters.. 82

Crunchy Kale Chips... 83

Vegan Taco Meat... 84

Baked Artichokes... 85

Tasty Broccoli Bites... 86

Baked Rainbow Fries.. 87

Vegan Pistachio Fudge Mini Cups.. 89

Baked Cheesy Mushrooms.. 90

Vegan Pumpkin Spice Crackers...92

Garlic Crackers with Thyme... 94

Avocado Fries.. 96

Tasty Apple Chips.. 98

Chapter 6 – Beverage and Dessert Recipes.. 99

Mint and Berry Spa Water.. 99

Apple and Carrot Juice.. 100

Celery Juice with Beet... 101

Hemp Protein Smoothie with Banana....................................... 102

Vanilla Cake in a Mug... 103

Almond Balls with Cacao... 104

Delish Apple Pie Tart.. 105

Strawberry Shortcake... 107

Choco-Creamy Pudding... 109

Pecan Pie Bites... 110

Strawberry Mousse... 111

Conclusion.. 112

What is Lectin?

Lectin is a protein of plant origin which is found in abundance in beans, legumes, eggplant, tomatoes and many other fruits and vegetables which we consume on a daily basis. This protein, when ingested binds to carbohydrates. Put in simpler terms, the sugar molecules which are found on all cells of the body are magnets for lectins. Depending upon the type of cell and the sugar to which lectin is attached, the effects of lectins on the body vary significantly. They range from beneficial effects like bone growth to disastrous impacts like autoimmune diseases.

Lectins are a boon to the plant family. Found abundantly in legumes, lectins help the plants to fight infections, utilize nitrogen by facilitating the attachment of rhizobia and promote the survival of seeds in the digestive tract of animals, including humans. However, our digestive systems lack the enzymes which help in breaking down lectins into simpler parts. As a result, they enter the bloodstream unchanged, causing some undesirable effects.

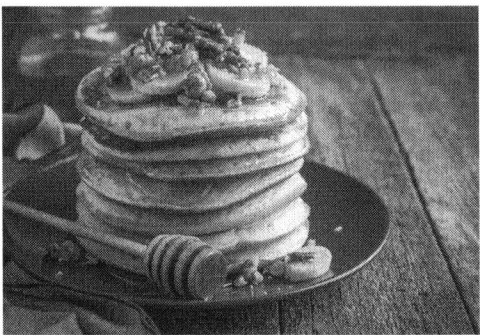

Due to extensive research in the realm of food and nutrition, health specialists and dieticians are now emphasizing on the elimination of lectin-rich foods from the diet. The effects have found to improve a lot in the overall health and in decreasing the incidence of lifestyle diseases, autoimmune diseases, and gastrointestinal problems.

Why has eliminating lectin from your diet become important?

After getting an idea about what is a lectin, let us understand in detail, the health issues which arise due to its consumption.

1. ***The gut feeling*** - Our stomach and intestines are the first line of defense when we ingest something bad. Just as they say that you should trust your gut feeling, you should be careful when you encounter symptoms like nausea, vomiting, diarrhea, flatulence, etc. These symptoms arise either due to excessive consumption of lectin or due to intolerance of the body to lectin-containing foods, which sometimes end up destroying the delicate intestinal lining. When this process keeps on happening without giving the gut, sufficient time to repair and regenerate, a condition known as 'Leaky gut' may arise. The useful molecules in our bodies may then find a way out via the stools giving rise to malnutrition, nutrient deficiencies, and many other complications.

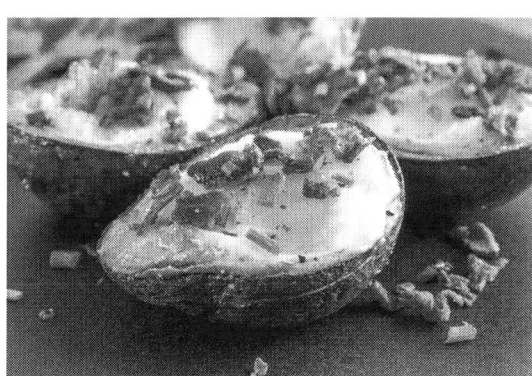

2. ***Autoimmunity*** - Our immune system is a mechanism of the body to fight and kill any microbes or harmful particles that may invade our body. However, in autoimmunity, the cells of the immune system begin to treat the healthy cells of the body

as the enemy. They start forming antibodies which in turn destroy these cells. Lectins are a huge culprit when it comes to triggering autoimmune responses in the body. These autoimmune disorders are often chronic, taking months and years to resolve. In worst case scenarios, they may even persist for a lifetime.
3. ***They assist in the infectious process*** - It has been found that many viruses including hepatitis C bind to lectins on the cell surface. To be exact, binding to lectins helps these viruses to invade and destroy the cells of the body leading to the development of deadly infections.
4. ***Other diseases*** - Some of the diseases which have been found to have an association with lectin ingestion include obesity, cardiovascular diseases, diabetes mellitus, arthritis, thyroid disorders and irritable bowel syndrome.

Foods containing Lectin

Some of the foods which are rich in lectin include:

a. ***Beans and Legumes*** - Out of all the food categories, beans and legumes are the richest in their lectin content. They are mainly concentrated in the cotyledon part of the seed. People who consume high amounts of legumes, especially when they are raw or improperly cooked are at high risk of developing diseases mentioned above.

b. ***Squash*** - This family of food, which mainly comprises of zucchini, pumpkin and squash host a lectin party in the seeds and the peel. For people who are fond of consuming these foods, make sure you remove all the seeds and peel the vegetable properly before consumption.

c. ***Tomatoes*** - Just like squash and zucchini, tomatoes have a good amount of lectin content in their seeds. Before you add tomatoes to your favorite dish, make sure to eliminate all the seeds and only use the juicy outer part of the fruit.

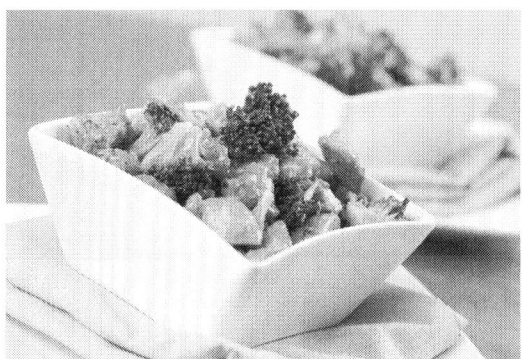

d. ***Grains*** - Scientific advancements and experiments are coming with many varieties of grains which are now fortified and processed to increase their nutritive value. But here is a bitter truth- more the processing, more will be the amount of lectin in the grains. If you are planning on eliminating lectins from your diet, you will have to go completely grain free.

e. *Peppers*- Many of us love the zing and spice that peppers add to our food. But unfortunately, these are a part of the list of foods containing lectin. Just like the others, lectins are mainly concentrated in the seeds. So if you love adding pepper to any food you eat, make sure to remove the seeds first.

f. *Corn*- After legumes, corn is ranked as one of the worst foods containing lectins. Eliminate any form of corn intake in your diet.

Choose the substitutes

Have you wondered, if we have to eliminate so many foods groups from our diet, where will we get the nutrition from? The vitamins and minerals supplied by these foods will no more find their way into our bodies leading to numerous deficiency diseases. Do not worry, because the substitutes for lectin-rich foods will efficiently replenish the nutrient reserves of your body without the unnecessary lectin exposure. Here are a few foods which you can use as substitutes for the foods mentioned above.

   a. ***Green leafy vegetables***- Not everybody's liking, but is a superfood when it comes to nutrition and benefits. Green leafy vegetables are packed with vitamins, minerals, and fiber. They are extremely beneficial to the body, boost the immune system, help the gut to function smoothly and also aid in losing weight when taken with salads and soup. Spinach, green lettuce, butter lettuce, kale, romaine, and parsley are excellent substitutes for beans and legumes.
   b. ***Tubers***- Elimination of grains leaves the body depleted of complex carbohydrates. Tubers like potato and sweet potato are a delicious way of adding these back in your diet. The good part is that you can use these tubers in many different dishes and delicacies. Not only carbohydrates, but tubers also enrich the body with micronutrients to keep it healthy and robust.

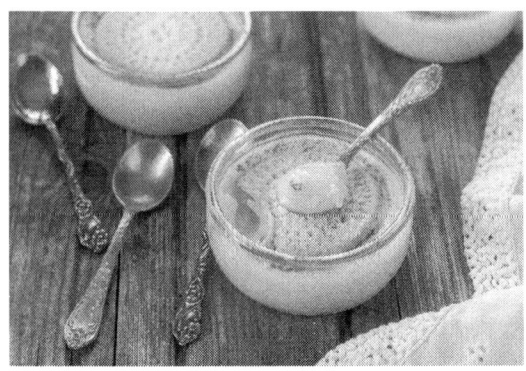

c. ***Time to go dairy free*** - While dairy may not have lectin as one of its major proteins, milk from some of the cows may be high in a protein known as casein A1, which structurally very similar to lectin and elicits a similar response in the body. If you know where your milk products are being produced and processes and you are assured that they are free of casein A1, then go ahead and relish the taste. However, if you have the slightest of doubt regarding the reliability of your dairy source, it is the best option to shift to dairy-free products. Coconut milk, almond milk and soy milk and substitutes for cow's milk with their nutritive value at par with that of cow's milk. With the rising trend of veganism, these are now readily available in the market.

d. ***Lectin free vegetables*** - Some of the nutritious vegetables which are free of lectin yet very nutritious include avocado, celery, cauliflower, garlic, onion and Brussel sprouts. They pair up well with well with any vegetable, and some of them can even be eaten raw, e.g., avocado.

Cooking and processing methods which help in reducing the quantity of lectin in diet

It may not be entirely possible to remove all the lectin-rich foods from the diet. However, before consumption, you can reduce the amount of lectin that enters into your stomach. Here are a few cooking techniques that you must employ for cooking lectin-rich foods.

   a. ***Boiling***- This is by far the easiest way to reduce the lectin content of foods. By boiling, the lectins bind to carbohydrates already present in the foods. As binding to carbohydrates helps in their faster elimination from the body without getting absorbed into the bloodstream.
   b. ***Cooking with the help of a pressure cooker-*** A pressure cooker very efficiently destroys plant lectins. It is the best option for foods which are high in their lectin content, e.g., beans and legumes. However, there is one significant drawback. Use of pressure cooker does not reduce the stubborn lectin content of grains like barley, rye, oats, and wheat.

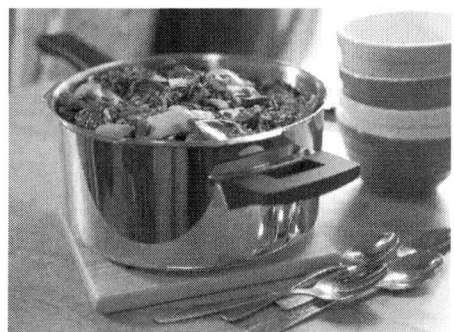

   c. ***Sprouting***- Since lectin is concerned with the preservation of seeds, sprouting them will eliminate enormous amounts of lectin which is stored within them. To sprout the grains, wrap them in a wet cloth or soak them in water overnight. Use these sprouts in your salads and soups for a much less lectin and much more nutrition.

d. ***Use the lectin-free part-*** Since the peel and seeds of veggies are the main part where the lectin resides, it is essential to remove these parts before consuming the vegetable.

e. ***Time to opt old school ways-*** In earlier times, the hull from the rice was separated, and the remaining white part was consumed. The techniques may have changed, but the idea behind it is still the same. For someone who consumes rice on a daily basis, it is advisable to use white rice instead of brown rice as the outer most part carries a lot of lectin content in it.

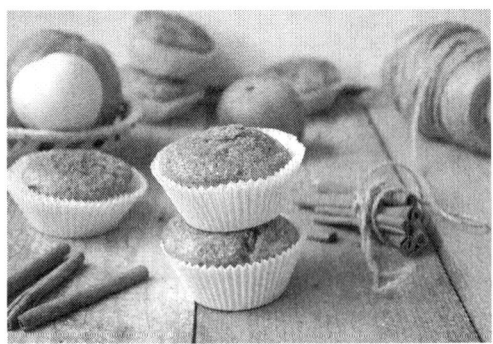

f. ***Brown bread may not be the healthiest-*** Almost every person is now switching to brown bread because it is considered as "healthier." However, just like brown rice, brown bread has a higher content of lectin that white bread. If you are looking to cut down on your lectin intake, switching your brown bread with the white one would be the next best step.

Say no to these foods

Shifting to a lectin free diet can be a considerable challenge. From changing your grocery lists to controlling your cravings, lectin free diets can test your patience in many different ways. To make things easier, we have prepared a simple list of foods which you have to avoid entirely. These include

- *Grains like wheat, barley, rye, oats*
- *Milk and milk products*
- *Corn*
- *Nightshade plants*
- *Sources of animal proteins like beef, pork, chicken*
- *Eggs*
- *Beans and Legumes*

Say yes to these foods

Here is a list of foods which you can now add to your grocery list to enjoy a hearty and a lectin free meal.

- *Cruciferous vegetables which include broccoli, cauliflower, and Brussel sprouts*
- *Kimchi*
- *Celery*
- *Avocado*
- *Artichokes*
- *Asparagus*
- *Mushrooms*
- *Fennel*
- *Red, green and butter lettuce*
- *Spinach*
- *Romaine*
- *Kale*
- *Kohlrabi*
- *Cilantro*
- *Beetroot*
- *Onion*
- *Arugula*

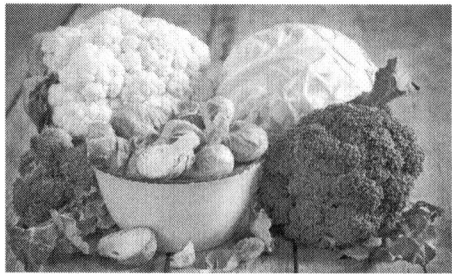

Use anti-inflammatory oils for cooking. These will soothe the lining of the intestines, help in its repair and also provide good fats to the body. These include- olive oil, avocado oil, coconut oil, sesame seed oil, flaxseed oil and macadamia nut oil.

For the touch of spices and seasoning, use lemon juice, vinegar, black pepper, mint leaves and freshly ground herbs and spices.

Take away message

Humans have been consuming lectin-rich foods for centuries. However, only with a thorough understanding and many experiments have the scientists been able to find out its implication in the causation of autoimmune and gastrointestinal diseases. Observe and understand the signs your body gives you. If you develop any gastric discomfort on consumption of legumes, grains, seeds, etc., it would be a good idea to start switching onto a lectin free diet. Since it is a significant lifestyle change, try to make a slow transition over a period of days to prevent you from falling back into the usual dietary patterns. You will soon begin to notice beautiful changes in your body. Your gut will function properly, you will start to lose weight, and the risk for cardiovascular and autoimmune diseases will fall tremendously.

Introduction

I want to thank you and congratulate you for downloading the book, "The Lectin Free Cookbook: Healthy, Yummy, and Lectin-Free Recipes that will Help You Lose Weight".

This book contains proven steps and strategies on how to prepare the best-tasting lectin-free recipes that will help you lose weight without needing to sacrifice a lot of your favorite foods. This kind of diet removes foods with high lectin content from your food list. They include eggplant, peppers, tomatoes, legumes, quinoa, and grains. You should also avoid conventionally-raised poultry and meat, out-of-season fruit, and dairy.

You will instead focus more on foods with low lectin content, such as wild-caught fish and pasture-raised meats. You can also indulge in nuts, seeds, mushrooms, asparagus, millet, broccoli, cauliflower, and more. It is ideal to use organic, homemade, and fresh ingredients.

How will you lose weight in this kind of diet? After eating the foods allowed in the diet, your body will no longer store fat like it used to. This book contains a variety of recipes that you can prepare throughout the day. The recipes are easy-to-follow and taste delicious. You will not notice that you are actually on a diet until you begin noticing that you are shedding off the unwanted pounds.

Chapter 1 – Salad Recipes

Roasted Artichoke Salad

Yield: 1 to 2 servings

Ingredients:

For the Seasoning

- 1/8 teaspoon ground paprika
- 1/8 teaspoon ground black pepper
- 1/8 teaspoon Himalayan pink salt
- 1/8 teaspoon ground garlic powder
- For the artichokes:
- 1 tablespoon avocado oil (100 percent pure)
- 1 14-ounce can artichoke hearts (drained)

For the vinaigrette

- 1 tablespoon date nectar
- 1/8 teaspoon black ground pepper
- 1 shallot (finely chopped)
- 1/8 teaspoon Himalayan pink salt
- 2 tablespoons avocado oil (100 percent pure)
- 1 tablespoon sesame seeds
- 2 tablespoons apple cider vinegar

For the salad

- 2 to 4 cups mixed salad greens

Directions:

1. Put all ingredients for the seasoning in a bowl. Mix well and set aside.

2. Chop off the tips of the artichokes and cut into smaller pieces. Put in a different bowl along with avocado oil. Toss to coat. Add the seasoning mix. Gently toss until combined.

3. Arrange the seasoned artichokes in a pan lined with parchment paper. Roast in a preheated oven at 425 degrees for 15 minutes. Toss the pieces and roast for 10 more minutes.

4. Put all ingredients for the vinaigrette in a bowl. Mix until combined. Adjust according to taste.

5. Arrange 2 handfuls of the salad greens in a platter. Add the roasted artichokes on top and drizzle with the vinaigrette.

6. Serve at once.

Salmon Salad with Orange and Cheese

Yield: 1 serving

Ingredients:

- 2 ounces real Feta cheese crumbles
- 2 Navel oranges (peeled and sectioned)
- 1 pound wild salmon flakes
- 1/3 cup chopped hazelnuts (toasted)
- 1 small red onion (sliced)
- 5 ounces baby spinach

For the Dijon Vinaigrette

- 4 tablespoons extra virgin olive oil
- 1 teaspoon Dijon mustard
- 1 teaspoon honey (optional)
- Salt to taste
- 1 tablespoon fresh dill (chopped)
- 3 tablespoons white wine vinegar
- 1 lemon (juiced)

Directions:

1. Toss all ingredients for the salad and arrange on a plate.

2. Put all ingredients for the vinaigrette in a bowl. Whisk until combined.

3. Drizzle salad with the vinaigrette before serving.

Sweet Potato Salad with Vegan Cilantro Pesto

Yield: 2 cups

Ingredients:

For the sweet potatoes

- Himalayan pink salt and ground black pepper to taste
- 2 cups organic sweet potatoes (peeled and cut into cubes)

For the cilantro pesto

- 3 tablespoons apple cider vinegar
- 3 garlic cloves
- 1/3 cup nutritional yeast
- 1/2 cup pine nuts
- 1/2 teaspoon ground black pepper
- 1/2 teaspoon Himalayan pink salt
- 1/2 cup extra virgin olive oil
- 2 cups fresh cilantro

Directions:

1. Arrange the potato cubes on a baking tray lined with parchment paper. Sprinkle with salt and pepper.

Bake in a preheated oven at 350 degrees for 35 minutes or until soft.

2. Put all liquid ingredients for the cilantro pesto in a blender. Process until combined. Add the remaining ingredients and process until smooth. Add seasonings according to taste.

3. Transfer the baked potatoes to a bowl. Add the pesto and toss until combined. Cover the bowl and refrigerate for at least 30 minutes before serving.

Kale Salad with Ham

Yield: 1 serving

Ingredients:

- 2 ounces Parmesan cheese (grated)
- 1 sweet onion (sliced)
- 1 bunch Lacinato kale (torn into smaller pieces)
- 1/4 cup pine nuts
- 2 ounces Spanish ham (diced)

For the lemon oil

- 2 tablespoons olive oil
- 1/2 lemon (juiced)
- Salt to taste

Directions:

1. Put all ingredients for the lemon oil in a bowl. Mix well and adjust according to taste.
2. Put all ingredients for the salad on a platter. Drizzle with lemon oil. Gently toss until combined.

Ham and Arugula Salad with Sweet Potato

Yield: 4 servings

Ingredients:

- 1/4 cup fresh tarragon leaves
- 2 ounces real Swiss cheese (shredded)
- 5 ounces baby arugula
- 1 pound sweet potato (peeled and cut into cubes)
- 1/4 cup shredded Parmesan cheese
- 2 ounces Prosciutto di Parma (crumbled)
- 1 tablespoon Dijon mustard
- 1 tablespoon white wine vinegar
- 1/4 cup extra virgin olive oil
- Sea salt and black pepper

Directions:

1. Put the sweet potatoes in a pot. Add enough cold water to cover all potatoes. Bring water to a boil over medium-high flame. Stir in 1 1/2 tablespoons of salt. Turn the heat to low and simmer for about 12 minutes.

2. Drain water from the pot. Rinse potatoes under cold water and dice into thin pieces.

3. Put half a teaspoon of salt, 1/4 teaspoon of pepper, mustard, vinegar, and oil in a bowl. Whisk until combined.

4. Divide the arugula into 4 small plates. Top each plate with sweet potatoes, tarragon, Swiss cheese, and ham. Add sauce and sprinkle with Parmesan cheese.

Steak Salad with Yogurt Dressing

Yield: 1 serving

Ingredients:

- 1 cup shirataki rice (rinsed and drained)
- 2 tablespoons pine nuts (toasted)
- 5 ounces baby spinach
- 1 pound medium-rare cooked grass-fed steak (sliced)

For the Yogurt Dressing

- 1 cup whole goat milk yogurt
- 2 teaspoons fresh thyme leaves
- 2 tablespoons red wine vinegar
- Salt and pepper to taste

Directions:

1. Put all ingredients for the yogurt dressing in a bowl. Whisk until combined.
2. Put all salad ingredients on a platter. Add the dressing. Toss until combined.

Peaches and Berries Salad with Spicy Tahini Dressing

Yield: 4 servings

Ingredients

For the Salad

- 1 cup   pecans
- 2 cups peaches (peeled and cubed)
- 2 cups blueberries
- 8 handfuls of spring salad mix

For the Tahini dressing

- 8 to 10 tablespoons purified water
- 1/2 teaspoon ground ginger
- 1/2 cup date nectar
- 1/2 cup tahini

Directions:

1. Put all ingredients for the tahini dressing in a bowl. Whisk until combined. Adjust water and sweetener according to taste.

2. Divide the spring salad mix into 4 bowls. Top each with pecans, peaches, and blueberries. Drizzle salad with the dressing before serving.

Shrimp Salad with Herbed Vinaigrette

Yield: 2 servings

Ingredients:

For the salad

- 1 bunch radishes (quartered)
- 1/2 red onion (thinly sliced)
- 1 head escarole (torn into bite-size pieces)
- 1 pound shrimp (cooked with tail-on)

For the herbed vinaigrette

- 1/4 cup extra virgin olive oil
- Salt and pepper to taste
- 2 tablespoons white wine vinegar
- 1 teaspoon Dijon mustard
- 2 tablespoons fresh chives (chopped)
- 2 garlic cloves (minced)
- 2 tablespoons capers
- 1 small shallot (minced)

Directions:

1. Put all ingredients for the salad in a bowl. Toss to combine.

2. Mix to combine all ingredients for the vinaigrette in a small bowl. Pour this on top of the salad. Toss the salad until combined.

3. Serve at once.

Sweet Potato with Chipotle Salad and Tahini Dressing

Yield: 1 to 2 servings

Ingredients:

- 2 tablespoons red onions (diced)
- 1 avocado (cubed)
- 2 handfuls spring salad mix

For the sweet potatoes

- 1/4 teaspoon Himalayan pink salt
- 1/2 teaspoon ground garlic powder
- 1 teaspoon ground chipotle powder
- 1 tablespoon avocado oil (100 percent pure)
- 2 cups organic sweet potato cubes (peeled and cubed)

For the tahini dressing

- 2 pinches ground black pepper
- 1/4 teaspoon Himalayan pink salt
- 1/4 teaspoon ground garlic powder
- 2 tablespoons filtered water
- 3 tablespoons lime juice
- 1/4 cup organic tahini

Directions:

1. Put the sweet potato cubes in a bowl along with avocado oil. Toss until combined.

2. In another bowl, stir to combine garlic powder, chipotle powder, and Himalayan pink salt.

3. Transfer the sweet potato cubes in a pan lined with parchment paper. Sprinkle with the seasoning mix. Bake in a preheated oven at 350 degrees for 25 minutes.

4. Put all ingredients for the dressing in a bowl. Whisk until combined. Adjust seasonings according to taste.

5. Arrange the spring salad mix in a platter. Top with cubed avocado and diced red onions. Add the baked potatoes and pour dressing all over the salad.

6. Serve while warm.

Chapter 2 – Vegan Ice Cream Recipes

Superfood Ice Cream with Cacao Nibs

Yield: 2 servings

Ingredients:

- 1 teaspoon baobab powder
- 2 teaspoons moringa powder
- 1/2 cup organic granular sweetener
- 1 13.5-ounce can full-fat coconut milk
- 1/2 cup raw cacao nibs (for the mix-in)

Directions:

1. Put all ingredients for the ice cream in a blender. Process until smooth and combined. Adjust sweetener according to taste.

2. Transfer mixture to an ice cream maker. Process according to package directions. Fold in the cacao nibs.

3. You can already enjoy this like a soft-serve ice cream. If you want it firmer, transfer to a container, cover, and freeze for at least an hour.

Chocolatey Avocado Ice Cream

Yield: 2 servings

Ingredients:

For the ice cream

- 1/4 cup Xylitol (non-GMO)
- 1/4 cup raw cacao powder
- 2 avocados (pitted)
- 1 13.5-ounce can full-fat coconut milk

For the swirl

- 1 tablespoon organic date nectar
- 1/2 cup almond butter

Directions:

1. Put all ingredients for the ice cream in a blender. Process until creamy. Adjust the sweetener according to taste. Transfer to an ice cream maker and process according to package directions.

2. Put all ingredients for the swirl in a bowl. Mix until combined. Set this aside.

3. Transfer ice cream to a container. Add a tablespoon of the swirl on top and swirl using the edge of a knife. Cover the container and freeze for at least 2 hours.

Cauli-Banana Ice Cream

Yield: 1 to 2 servings

Ingredients:

For the ice cream

- 1 tablespoon almond butter
- 2 tablespoons raw cacao powder
- 1/4 cup, plus 1 tablespoon homemade almond milk
- 1 cup cauliflower rice (frozen)
- 1 large banana (frozen)

For the toppings

- 1 to 2 tablespoons raw cacao nibs
- 1/2 cup wild blueberries

Directions:

1. Put all ingredients for the ice cream in a blender. Process on a high speed until the consistency is similar to a soft-serve ice cream. Transfer to bowls. Top with blueberries and cacao nibs and serve at once.

Vegan Vanilla Ice Cream
Yield: 2 to 4 servings

Ingredients:

- 2 teaspoons vanilla extract
- 2 13.5-ounce cans full-fat coconut milk
- 1/2 cup Stevia blend (non-GMO)
- 1 pinch Himalayan pink salt
- 1 teaspoon vanilla bean powder

Directions:

1. Put all ingredients in a blender and process until combined. Transfer mixture to an ice cream machine. Process according to package directions.

2. Transfer to a container, cover, and freeze for at least 2 hours before serving. If you don't want to wait, you can enjoy it as a soft serve ice cream directly from the machine.

Strawberry Ice Cream

Yield: 4 servings

Ingredients:

- 2 cups diced strawberries

For the ice cream

- 2 teaspoons organic pure vanilla extract
- 1/2 cup Xylitol (non-GMO)
- 2 13.5-ounce cans organic full-fat coconut milk

Directions:

1. Put all ingredients for the ice cream in a blender and process until smooth. Adjust sweetener according to taste. Transfer to an ice cream machine and process according to package directions.
2. Transfer processed ice cream to a container. Fold in the diced strawberries. Cover the container and freeze for a couple of hours before serving.

Avocado and Raspberry Ice Cream Squares

Yield: 12 small squares

Ingredients:

- 1 cup freeze-dried raspberries for add-ins, plus 1/2 cup for toppings

For the ice cream

- 1/4 teaspoon Himalayan pink salt
- 1/4 teaspoon vanilla bean powder
- 1/4 cup organic date nectar
- 1/2 cup raw cacao powder
- 1 13.5-ounce can full-fat coconut milk
- 2 organic avocados (pitted)

Directions:

1. Freeze the can of coconut milk an hour before making the ice cream. Scoop the hardened fat and put in a blender. Reserve the remaining water from the can for a smoothie or other recipes. Add the rest of the ingredients for the ice cream to the blender and process until smooth. Add a cup of the free-dried raspberries and manually fold them into the mixture.

2. Transfer to an 8 by 5 pan lined with parchment paper. Use a spatula to spread it evenly. Add the toppings and freeze for 3 hours.

3. Once the ice cream is set, slice into squares. Put them in a container and freeze until ready to serve.

Chapter 3 – Breakfast Recipes

Cheesy Breakfast Burritos

Yield: 4 servings

Ingredients:

- 8 cassava flour tortillas (around 6 inches)
- 4 ounces crumbled goat cheese
- 6 eggs (beaten)
- Himalayan sea salt and black pepper to taste
- 2 garlic cloves (sliced)
- 2 ounces chopped spinach
- 2 tablespoons extra virgin olive oil

Directions:

1. Heat oil in a pan over medium flame. Add spinach, 1/4 teaspoon pepper, half a teaspoon of salt, and garlic. Stir until combined. Leave to cook for 3 minutes. Add the eggs all over the spinach. Leave to rest for 30 seconds. Using a spatula, push the eggs around the pan for about 4 minutes or until cooked. Remove from the stove. Put goat cheese on top and leave to soften.

2. Cover 4 tortillas at a time with a moist paper towel and heat in the microwave for 30 seconds.

3. Divide the cooked eggs into the heated tortillas. Fold each piece like a taco and serve while warm.

Flourless Garlic Breadsticks

Yield: 12 breadsticks

Ingredients:

For the garlic topping

- 1/8 teaspoon ground black pepper
- 1/8 teaspoon Himalayan pink salt
- 1 tablespoon dried oregano
- 1 tablespoon extra virgin olive oil
- 4 garlic cloves (crushed)

For the breadsticks

- 3 flax eggs (combination of 9 tablespoons of filtered water and 3 tablespoons ground flax seeds)
- 1/2 teaspoon Himalayan pink salt
- 1 teaspoon ground garlic powder
- 1 teaspoon extra virgin olive oil
- 2 cups mozzarella cheese
- 2 cups almond flour

Directions:

1. Put all ingredients for the breadsticks in a bowl. Mix until combined. Using your hands, shape the mixture

into a ball. Put it on a pan lined with parchment paper and flatten out with about half an inch thickness. Bake in a preheated oven at 350 degrees for 20 minutes.

2. Put all ingredients for the garlic topping in a bowl. Mix until combined. Adjust seasonings according to taste. Spread the topping all over the baked bread.

3. Slice the bread into bite-size pieces and immediately serve.

Shirataki Fettuccine Pasta with Artichoke and Basil

Yield: 2 to 4 servings

Ingredients:

- 2 packs Shirataki Fettuccine Pasta
- For the sauce
- 1/2 teaspoon ground black pepper
- 1/2 teaspoon Himalayan pink salt
- 1 tablespoon extra virgin olive oil
- 2 garlic cloves (crushed)
- 2 tablespoons nutritional yeast
- 2 tablespoons freshly squeezed lemon juice
- 3/4 cup homemade almond milk
- 1 1/4 cups pine nuts
- For add-ins
- 1 14-ounce can artichoke hearts (chopped into long strips)
- 8 leaves fresh basil (chopped)

Directions:

1. Cook noodles according to package directions. Set aside.

2. Put all ingredients for the sauce in a blender. Process until combined and smooth. Adjust seasonings according to taste.

3. Put the cooked noodles and add-ins in a bowl. Add the sauce and gently toss until combined. Top with extra chopped basil before serving.

Protein Energy Balls with Dried Blueberries

Yield: 12 balls

Ingredients:

- 1 teaspoon vanilla bean powder
- 1 tablespoon almond butter
- 1 cup Medjool dates (pitted)
- 1 cup dried blueberries
- 2 tablespoons lectin-free protein powder

Directions:

1. Put all ingredients in a food processor. Pulse about 10 times. Get a spoonful of the mixture at a time and form it into a ball using your hands. Arrange the balls on a container. Cover and refrigerate for at least 30 minutes before serving.

Cauliflower Risotto with Mushrooms

Yield: 2 cups

Ingredients:

- 1/2 teaspoon ground sage
- 1 teaspoon ground black pepper
- 1 teaspoon Himalayan pink salt
- 2 tablespoons extra virgin olive oil
- 2 garlic cloves (crushed)
- 1/2 cup red onion (diced)
- 1 1/2 cups baby bella mushrooms (diced)
- For add-ins:
- 4 cups cauliflower rice
- 1 13.5-ounce can full-fat coconut milk

Directions:

1. Refrigerate the can of coconut milk the night before cooking the dish.
2. Put all ingredients in a pan, except the coconut milk and cauliflower rice, over medium-high flame. Saute for 5 minutes.
3. Scoop out the hardened coconut fat from the can. Reserve the liquid for other recipes. Transfer the

coconut fat to the pan and add the cauliflower rice. Stir to combine all ingredients. Turn the heat to medium and simmer until the cauliflower rice becomes soft. Adjust seasonings according to taste.

4. Serve while hot.

Tasty Mushroom Soup
Yield: 2 to 4 servings

Ingredients:

- 1 garlic clove (crushed)
- 1 13.5-ounce can full-fat coconut milk
- 1 cup vegetable broth
- 1/2 cup red onions (chopped)
- 1/2 teaspoon dried thyme
- 1/2 teaspoon ground black pepper
- 1/2 teaspoon Himalayan pink salt
- 2 teaspoons avocado oil (100 percent pure)
- 1 tablespoon coconut aminos
- 1 cup baby bella mushrooms (diced)
- 1 cup shitake mushrooms (diced)

Directions:

1. Heat avocado oil in a pan over medium-high flame. Add the onions, garlic, mushrooms, dried thyme, black pepper, and Himalayan salt. Saute for 3 minutes. Add the coconut aminos, coconut milk, and vegetable broth. Stir until combined. Adjust seasonings according to taste. Turn the heat to

medium-low and simmer for 15 minutes while stirring occasionally.

2. Top with chopped green onions, sliced mushrooms, and a bit of ground black pepper before serving.

Baked Peach Cobbler Pancakes

Yield: 4 servings

Ingredients:

- 2 ripe peaches (peeled and thinly sliced)
- 1/4 teaspoon baking soda
- 1/2 teaspoon baking powder
- 1/4 teaspoon sea salt
- 1/4 cup cassava flour
- 1/4 cup tapioca flour
- 1/4 cup coconut flour
- 1 tablespoon coconut oil (melted)
- 5 ounces goat milk kefir
- 5 drops liquid stevia
- Cinnamon (for sprinkling)
- 1 teaspoon vanilla extract
- 2 large pastured eggs

Directions:

1. In a bowl, put the eggs, kefir, stevia, and vanilla. Whisk until combined. Continue whisking as you

gradually add the coconut oil to make sure that it doesn't solidify.

2. In another bowl, put the baking powder, sea salt, cassava flour, tapioca flour, and coconut flour. Mix until combined. Add this to the wet mixture. Whisk batter until smooth.

3. Transfer batter to a greased pie pan. Add half of the peaches on top and sprinkle with cinnamon. Bake in a preheated oven at 350 degrees for 30 minutes. Leave to cool for a few minutes before adding the remaining peaches on top. Serve while warm.

Cassava Flour Pancakes with Cinnamon

Yield: 4 servings

Ingredients:

- 1/4 cup water
- 3 tablespoons melted butter, plus more for serving
- 2 eggs (room temperature)
- 1/2 teaspoon vanilla extract
- 1 teaspoon cinnamon, plus more for serving
- 1 tablespoon baking powder
- 2 tablespoons monk's fruit sweetener
- 1 1/4 cup goat milk kefir
- 1/8 teaspoon nutmeg
- 1/4 teaspoon sea salt
- 1 cup cassava flour

Directions:

1. In a bowl, whisk to combine the dry ingredients – nutmeg, sea salt, cinnamon, baking powder, sweetener, and flour.
2. Put the wet ingredients in another bowl – eggs, vanilla, water, and kefir. Whisk until combined. Gradually whisk butter into the mixture.

3. Combine the 2 mixtures and whisk unto smooth.

4. Cook 3 pancakes in a nonstick pan over medium-low flame at a time. Transfer to a plate. Add butter and cinnamon on top before serving.

Cream of Asparagus Soup

Yield: 4 cups

Ingredients:

For add-ins

- 1 13.5-ounce can organic full-fat coconut milk
- 1 cup vegetable broth

For the sauteed vegetables

- 2 teaspoons organic extra-virgin olive oil
- 3 garlic cloves (crushed)
- 1 cup onion (diced)
- 12 stalks of asparagus (chopped)
- Himalayan pink salt and ground pepper to taste

Directions:

1. Heat olive oil in a skillet over medium-high flame. Add garlic, onions, asparagus, black pepper, and salt. Saute for 4 to 5 minutes. Adjust the seasonings according to taste.

2. Pour the coconut milk and vegetable broth on a blender. Add the cooked vegetables. Process on a high-speed setting until smooth and creamy. Transfer to a saucepan over medium flame. Simmer until warm.

Cauli Rice with Lime

Yield: 1 1/2 cups

Ingredients:

- 1/4 cup fresh cilantro (chopped)

For the cauliflower rice

- 1/2 teaspoon ground black pepper
- 1 teaspoon Himalayan pink salt
- 1 tablespoon avocado oil (100 percent pure)
- 2 tablespoons lime juice
- 2 cups cauliflower rice

Directions:

1. Put all ingredients for the cauliflower rice in a pan over medium-high flame. Toss until combined. Adjust seasonings according to taste and saute for 5 minutes. Remove from the stove. Stir in the chopped cilantro.

2. Transfer to a platter. Top with extra chopped cilantro before serving.

Chapter 4 – Main Course Recipes

Cheesy Chicken Enchiladas with Adobo Sauce

Yield: 8 enchiladas

Ingredients:

- 4 garlic cloves (peeled)
- 8 ounces crumbled goat cheese
- Sea salt and black pepper to taste
- 2 cups broth (divided)
- 8 ounces cooked pastured chicken (shredded)
- 1 white onion (chopped)
- 8 ounces shiitake mushrooms (chopped)
- 2 tablespoons olive oil
- Hot sauce and chopped fresh cilantro (for serving)
- 8 cassava flour tortillas (warmed in the microwave)
- 1/4 teaspoon paprika
- 1/2 teaspoon dried oregano
- 1/2 teaspoon ground cumin
- 1 teaspoon granular sweetener
- 1 teaspoon coconut aminos
- 3 teaspoons apple cider vinegar

Directions:

1. Heat oil in a pan over medium-high flame. Stir in the onions and mushrooms. Cook for about 8 minutes while constantly stirring. Add 1/4 teaspoon of pepper, half a teaspoon of salt, half a cup of broth, and chicken. Saute for a couple of minutes. Turn the heat to medium. Simmer for 4 minutes while stirring often.

2. Transfer the cooked dish to a bowl and add half of the crumbled goat cheese.

3. Prepare the adobo sauce. Put the remaining broth in a blender. Add coconut aminos, cider vinegar, paprika, oregano, cumin, sweetener, and 2 teaspoons of sea salt. Process for 3 minutes or until smooth. Pour half of the adobo sauce mixture into a glass baking dish.

4. Fill each tortilla with 1/4 cup of the mushroom mixture. Roll up and arrange all filled tortillas in the baking dish with the seam-side facing down. Drizzle the rest of the adobo sauce and goat cheese on top of the tortillas. Bake in a preheated oven at 350 degrees for 15 minutes.

5. Top with hot sauce and cilantro before serving.

Yummy Salmon Cakes

Yield: 4 servings

Ingredients:

- 2 scallions (roughly chopped)
- Sea salt and black pepper
- 2 tablespoons extra virgin olive oil (divided)
- 1/4 cup fresh mint (torn)
- 1/2 cup kalamata olives
- 1 cup millet
- 2 tablespoons Dijon mustard, plus more for serving
- 2 cups vegetable broth
- 1 pound wild Alaskan sockeye salmon (skinned)

Directions:

1. Put broth and millet in a saucepan over medium-high flame. Bring to a boil. Reduce flame to low, cover the pan, and simmer for 20 minutes. Stir in half a teaspoon of salt and pepper, a tablespoon of olive oil, mint, and olives.

2. Put salmon in a paper towel and squeeze out excess liquid. Transfer to a blender and add 1/4 teaspoon of pepper, half a teaspoon of salt, and scallions. Pulse until chopped. Transfer to a bowl. Add mustard and

half a cup of the cooked millet. Mix using your hands and form into 8 patties.

3. Heat a tablespoon of oil in a pan over medium flame. Cook the patties until both sides are browned. Transfer to a platter. Add some steamed greens and the remaining millet before serving.

Shirataki Angel Hair Pasta with Avocado Sauce

Yield: 2 servings

Ingredients:

- 2 packs Shirataki Angel Hair Pasta

For the sauce

- 1/2 teaspoon Himalayan pink salt
- 1 teaspoon ground chipotle powder
- 2 tablespoons lime juice
- 1/4 cup extra virgin olive oil
- 2 organic avocados

Directions:

1. Cook the pasta according to package directions.
2. Put all ingredients for the sauce in a blender. Process until smooth and creamy. Adjust the seasonings according to taste.
3. Put the cooked pasta in a bowl, add the sauce, and toss until combined. Top with chopped fresh cilantro and serve while warm.

Chicken Strips with Cilantro Dipping Sauce

Yield: 1 serving

Ingredients:

- 1/4 teaspoon sea salt
- 1/4 cup extra virgin olive oil
- 2 cups cilantro (chopped)
- 1 pastured chicken cutlet (sliced into strips)
- 1 tablespoon avocado oil

Directions:

1. Heat avocado oil in a pan over medium-high flame. Put the meat and sprinkle with salt. Stir for 4 minutes. Transfer to a platter and leave to cool.
2. Put sea salt, olive oil, and cilantro in a blender. Process on a high-speed setting until smooth.
3. Serve warm chicken strips with the dipping sauce on the side.

Cauli Rice with Basil Pesto

Yield: 2 cups

Ingredients:

For the cauliflower rice

- 1/2 teaspoon organic ground black pepper
- 1/2 teaspoon Himalayan pink salt
- 2 cloves organic garlic (freshly crushed)
- 1 tablespoon organic extra-virgin olive oil
- 1/2 cup organic red onions (diced)
- 4 cups organic cauliflower rice

For the basil pesto

- 1/2 teaspoon Himalayan pink salt
- 2 tablespoons lemon juice
- 1/4 cup extra virgin olive oil
- 1/4 cup nutritional yeast
- 1/2 cup walnuts
- 4 cups fresh basil
- 1/4 teaspoon ground black pepper

Directions:

1. Put all ingredients for the basil pesto in a blender. Process until combined and thick. Adjust seasonings according to taste.

2. Put all ingredients for the cauliflower rice in a pan over medium-high flame. Saute until cooked. Stir in the pesto mixture. Season with salt and pepper. Transfer to bowls and serve while warm.

Veggie-Filled Fettuccine Alfredo

Yield: 4 to 6 servings

Ingredients:

- 1/2 teaspoon Italian seasoning
- 1/4 cup Parmesan cheese (grated)
- 1 bunch thin asparagus (trimmed)
- 1/4 cup extra virgin olive oil, plus more for tossing
- Sea salt and black pepper
- 1/2 lemon (zested)
- 1/2 cup basil leaves or fresh Italian parsley (chopped)
- 1 cup mascarpone cheese
- 5 ounces shiitake mushrooms (sliced)
- 4 servings grain-free fettuccine pasta

Directions:

1. Cook pasta. Reserve a cup of the cooking liquid and strain pasta in a colander. Add some extra virgin olive oil and toss.

2. Heat a couple of tablespoons of olive oil in a pan over medium flame. Put the mushrooms, turn the heat to medium-high, and leave for 2 minutes. Stir and cook for 2 more minutes. Add the rest of olive oil, half a

teaspoon of salt, and asparagus. Cook for 3 minutes while stirring often. Remove from the stove. Add the cooked noodles and mascarpone cheese. Toss until combined. Gradually add the reserved cooking liquid until you have achieved the desired consistency for the sauce. Add lemon zest, Italian seasoning, herbs, and pecorino. Gently stir until combined.

3. Transfer to a platter. Season with salt and pepper and serve at once.

Baked Okra Bites

Yield: 2 to 4 servings

Ingredients:

- 2 tablespoons avocado oil (100 percent pure)
- 12 organic okra pods (sliced)

For the bread crumbs:

- 1/4 teaspoon Himalayan pink salt
- 1/4 teaspoon ground cayenne pepper
- 1/4 teaspoon ground garlic powder
- 1/4 cup nutritional yeast
- 1/4 cup almond flour

Directions:

1. Put all ingredients for the bread crumbs in a bowl and mix until combined.

2. Put the okra slices in another bowl along with a tablespoon of avocado oil. Toss until combined. Add half of the bread crumb mixture. Gently toss to coat. Add the rest of the avocado oil and bread crumb mixture. Gently toss to coat.

3. Arrange the coated okra slices in a pan lined with parchment paper. Bake in a preheated oven at 425

degrees for 12 minutes. Flip the okra pieces and bake for 8 more minutes.

4. Serve at once.

Vegan Fudgy Tarts

Yield: 3 tarts

Ingredients:

For the crust

- 1 pinch Himalayan pink salt
- 1 tablespoon organic coconut oil
- 1 cup organic medjool dates (pitted)
- 1 cup organic walnuts

For the filling

- 1 pinch Himalayan pink salt
- 1/4 cup raw cacao powder
- 1/2 cup date nectar
- 1/2 cup coconut oil
- 1/2 cup almond butter

Directions:

1. Put all ingredients for the crust in a food processor. Process until crumbly and wet. Divide the crust mixture into 3 tart molds. Use your finger of the back of a spoon to press the mixture at the bottom and sides of each mold. Set aside.

2. Put all ingredients for the filling in a bowl and whisk until smooth. Scoop filling into the molds. Refrigerate for 2 hours until firm.

3. Remove tarts from the molds and serve immediately.

Baked Sweet Potato Toast
Yield: 4 to 6 slices

Ingredients:

For the toast

- 1 to 2 teaspoons avocado oil (100 percent pure)
- 1 large sweet potato

For the guacamole

- 1/4 teaspoon Himalayan pink salt
- 1 to 2 pinches black ground pepper
- 1 teaspoon freshly squeezed lime juice
- 1 organic jalapeno (diced)
- 2 garlic cloves (crushed)
- 1 tablespoon chopped cilantro
- 1 tablespoon diced red onion
- 2 avocados

Directions:

1. Chop off the ends of the sweet potato. Slice into 1/4-inch thickness and put in a tray lined with parchment paper. Brush the sweet potato slices with a bit of avocado oil. Bake in a preheated oven at 350 degrees

for 25 minutes. Flip the potato slices and bake for 20 more minutes.

2. Put all ingredients for the guacamole in a bowl. Mash until combined. Add seasonings according to taste.

3. Put the sweet potato toast on a plate, top with guacamole sauce, and serve.

Walnut Fudge
Yield: 8 bars

Ingredients:

- 1/4 cup date nectar
- 1 teaspoon vanilla bean powder
- 1/4 cup chopped walnuts
- 1/4 cup almond butter
- 1/4 cup raw cacao powder
- 1 cup melted coconut oil

Directions:

1. Put all ingredients in a bowl and mix until smooth. Transfer to a bread pan and spread evenly all over. Freeze for an hour or until ready to serve.
2. Slice and serve.

Tasty Gingerbread in a Mug

Yield: 1 serving

Ingredients:

- 1 egg (lightly beaten)
- 1/2 tablespoon water
- 1/2 teaspoon apple cider vinegar
- 2 teaspoons Erythritol syrup (maple-flavored)
- 1/2 teaspoon baking powder
- 1/4 teaspoon cinnamon
- 1/2 teaspoon ground ginger
- 1 tablespoon cassava flour
- 1 tablespoon coconut flour
- 1 tablespoon butter (room temperature)
- Nutmeg, cloves, and allspice to taste

Directions:

1. Put the flours, butter, baking powder, allspice, cinnamon, and ginger in a heat-proof mug. Mix well. Add egg, cider vinegar, and syrup. Beat until combined. Scrape the sides and bottom of the mug. Continue mixing until the batter is smooth.

2. Microwave for 1 1/2 minutes. Add cinnamon and butter on top before serving.

Ravioli with Basil Pesto

Yield: 10 ravioli

Ingredients:

For serving

- 5 ounces mixed salad greens
- Balsamic vinegar and olive oil

For the ravioli

- 2 large pastured eggs (beaten with a teaspoon of water)
- 5 square coconut wraps
- 1/4 cup Parmesan cheese (grated)
- 1/4 cup mascarpone cheese
- 1 10-ounce package frozen spinach (thawed, squeezed dry, and chopped)
- 4 tablespoons extra virgin olive oil (divided)

For the basil pesto

- 1/2 cup extra virgin olive oil
- 2 garlic cloves
- 1 ounce crumbled Parmesan cheese
- 1/4 cup pine nuts
- 2 cups packed fresh basil

Directions:

1. Heat 2 tablespoons of oil in a pan over medium-high flame. Put the spinach and leave to cook for a couple of minutes. Transfer to a bowl. Add Parmesan cheese and mascarpone cheese. Gently stir until combined.

2. Spread 2 1/2 wraps on a chopping board. Brush them with the egg and water mixture. Put 1 tablespoon of the cheese and spinach mixture in each corner of the wrap. Brush another wrap with the egg mixture, put on top of the filling as you press and seal the ends. Slice to make ravioli squares. Cover with a clean cloth and leave to rest.

3. Put all ingredients for the basil pesto in a blender. Process until smooth.

4. Heat 2 tablespoons of olive oil in a pan over medium flame. Fry the ravioli in batches for around 3 minutes.

5. Arrange salad greens on a platter. Add the fried ravioli and pesto. Drizzle with balsamic vinegar before serving.

Chapter 5 – Soup and Appetizer Recipes

Mint and Berry Soup

Yield: 1 to 2 servings

Ingredients:

For the sweetener

- 1/4 cup Xylitol (non-GMO)
- 1/4 cup filtered water

For the soup

- 8 fresh mint leaves
- 1 teaspoon freshly squeezed lemon juice
- 1/2 cup filtered water
- 1 cup frozen mixed berries (blackberries, blueberries, raspberries)

Directions:

1. Heat water in a pan over low heat. Add sugar and stir until dissolved. Turn off the heat and leave to cool.

2. Pour the sweetener mixture on a blender and add all ingredients for the soup. Process until combined. Strain mixture to remove the seeds. Reserve seeds for a smoothie recipe.

3. Transfer soup to a bowl. Refrigerate for at least 30 minutes before serving.

Spiced Cauliflower Rice Soup

Yield: 4 cups

Ingredients:

- 1 13.5-ounce can full-fat coconut milk
- 1/2 teaspoon ground black pepper
- 1 teaspoon Himalayan pink salt
- 1 teaspoon dried rosemary
- 2 teaspoons pumpkin spice
- 2 tablespoons extra virgin olive oil
- 1 garlic clove (crushed)
- 1/2 cup diced red onion
- 4 cups cauliflower rice

Directions:

1. Heat oil in a pan over medium flame. Add garlic, onions, rosemary, salt, and pepper. Saute for 3 minutes. Add the pumpkin spice, coconut milk, and cauliflower rice. Mix well. Add more seasonings according to taste. Turn the heat to medium-low and simmer until cooked.

2. Transfer to a bowl. Sprinkle with a bit of pepper and dried rosemary and serve while hot.

Swiss Chard Fritters

Yield: 4 servings

Ingredients:

- 1/2 cup cassava flour
- 2 ounces goat cheese (crumbled)
- Sea salt and black pepper to taste
- 1/2 teaspoon ground cumin
- 3 garlic cloves (chopped)
- 1 bunch of Swiss chard (stemmed and torn into bite-size pieces)
- Sour cream (for serving)
- 4 tablespoons extra virgin olive oil (divided)

Directions:

1. Put Swiss chard, cumin, garlic, 1/4 teaspoon of pepper, and half a teaspoon of salt on a blender. Pulse until combined. Transfer mixture to a bowl. Add flour and goat cheese. Mix until combined.
2. Divide the mixture into 4 and form each into a patty with a 1/4-inch thickness.
3. Heat oil in a pan over medium-high flame. Cook the patties until both sides are browned. Transfer to a plate and serve along with a dollop of sour cream.

Crunchy Kale Chips

Yield: 2 to 4 servings

Ingredients:

- 1/2 teaspoon Himalayan pink salt
- 2 tablespoons nutritional yeast
- 1 tablespoon avocado oil (100 percent pure)
- 10 cups organic kale (stemmed and broken into bite-size pieces)

Directions:

1. Put kale and avocado oil in a bowl. Toss until combined. Sprinkle with salt and nutritional yeast. Use your hands to mix. Add more seasonings if preferred.   Transfer to a baking sheet lined with parchment paper and spread them all over. Bake in a preheated oven at 350 degrees for 8 minutes. Flip the pieces and continue baking for 8 more minutes.

Vegan Taco Meat

Yield: 1 1/2 cups

Ingredients:

- 1 teaspoon chili powder
- 1 teaspoon chipotle powder
- 1 teaspoon cumin powder
- 1/2 teaspoon Himalayan pink salt
- 10 teaspoons extra-virgin olive oil
- 2 cups walnuts

Directions:

1. Put all ingredients in a food processor and process until chopped. Put more seasonings if preferred.
2. Use the mixture as filling for taco or wrap or as topping for salad.

Baked Artichokes

Yield: 2 to 4 serving

Ingredients:

- 1 tablespoon avocado oil (100 percent pure)
- 1 can artichoke hearts (drained)

For the seasoning

- 1/2 teaspoon Himalayan pink salt
- 1/2 teaspoon ground cayenne pepper
- 1/2 teaspoon ground garlic
- 1/2 cup nutritional yeast
- 1/2 cup almond flour

Directions:

1. Put all ingredients for the seasoning in a bowl. Mix until combined.
2. Chop off the ends of the artichokes and slice each piece into 2. Tear leaves into smaller pieces. Put in a bowl along with avocado oil and half of the seasoning mixture. Toss until combined.
3. Transfer the seasoned artichokes to a pan lined with parchment paper. Spread them all over and sprinkle with the remaining seasoning mixture. Bake in a preheated oven at 425 degrees for 15 minutes.
4. Serve at once.

Tasty Broccoli Bites

Yield: 3 cups

Ingredients:

- 2 tablespoons avocado oil (100 percent pure)
- 3 cups organic broccoli florets

For the seasoning

- 1/4 teaspoon Himalayan pink salt
- 1/4 teaspoon ground cayenne pepper
- 1/4 teaspoon ground garlic powder
- 1/4 cup nutritional yeast
- 1/4 cup almond flour

Directions:

1. Put all ingredients for the seasoning in a bowl. Mix until combined. Add more seasonings according to taste.

2. Put the broccoli florets and avocado oil in a bowl. Toss until combined. Add half of the seasoning mixture and gently toss to coat. Transfer to a pan lined with parchment paper. Bake in a preheated oven at 400 degrees for 10 minutes. Transfer to a bowl and add the remaining seasoning mixture. Toss to coat. Put back to the pan and bake for 25 more minutes.

Baked Rainbow Fries

Yield: 8 servings

Ingredients:

- 3 tablespoons grainy mustard
- 3/4 cup full-fat sour cream
- Black pepper to taste
- 2 teaspoons sea salt
- 2 teaspoons granulated garlic
- 3 tablespoons extra virgin olive oil
- 2 medium sweet potatoes (peeled and sliced into strips)
- 2 medium yuca roots (peeled and sliced into strips)
- 4 purple carrots (peeled and sliced into strips)

Directions:

1. Put sweet potatoes, yucca roots, carrots, black pepper, salt, and granulated garlic in a bowl. Gently toss to coat.

2. Preheat two baking sheets in an oven at 450 degrees. Divide the seasoned rainbow fries into the 2 baking sheets. Place the sheets at the bottom thirds and top of the oven. Bake for 10 minutes. Toss the fries and continue baking for 10 more minutes.

3. In a small bowl, mix to combine the mustard and sour cream. Season with pepper.

4. Transfer fries in a bowl and serve with the dip.

Vegan Pistachio Fudge Mini Cups

Yield: 24 pieces

Ingredients:

- Sea salt as topping

For the fudge

- 1 teaspoon vanilla bean powder
- 1/4 cup almond butter
- 1/4 cup organic date nectar
- 1/4 cup raw cacao powder
- 1 cup melted coconut oil
- 1 cup chopped pistachios

Directions:

1. Put all ingredients for the fudge in a bowl. Mix well until smooth. Scoop batter into 24 mini muffin cups. Arrange cups on a tray and freeze for 10 minutes.
2. Sprinkle each cup with sea salt. Freeze for an hour before serving.

Baked Cheesy Mushrooms

Yield: 1 to 2 servings

Ingredients:

- 1 cup homemade almond milk
- 2 cups baby bella mushrooms (stemmed and sliced)

For the seasoning

- 1/2 teaspoon Himalayan pink salt
- 1/2 teaspoon ground garlic powder
- 1/2 teaspoon ground cayenne pepper
- 1/2 cup nutritional yeast
- 1/2 cup almond flour

Directions:

1. Put all ingredients for the seasoning in a bowl. Mix until combined. Add more salt, garlic, and pepper if preferred. You can use less of the cayenne pepper if you don't want the mixture to be too spicy.

2. Put half of the seasoning mixture in a bowl and almond milk in another bowl.

3. Soak a cup of mushroom in the bowl of milk. Toss until coated. Use a fork to transfer the mushrooms to the bowl of seasoning mixture. Gently toss to coat. Transfer to a baking tray lined with parchment paper

and spread all over. Repeat the same sequence to the rest of the mushrooms.

4. Bake in a preheated oven at 425 degrees for 12 minutes. Remove trays from the oven and flip the mushrooms. Continue baking for 8 more minutes.

5. Serve while hot.

Vegan Pumpkin Spice Crackers

Yield: Up to 35 crackers

Ingredients:

- Sea salt for topping

For the crackers

- 1/8 teaspoon ground garlic powder
- 1/4 teaspoon ground black pepper
- 1/2 teaspoon Himalayan pink salt
- 2 teaspoons pumpkin spice
- 1 flax egg (combination of 1 tablespoon of ground flax and 3 tablespoons of filtered water)
- 1 tablespoon avocado oil (100 percent pure)
- 2 cups almond flour

Directions:

1. Put all ingredients for the crackers in a bowl. Mix until combined.
2. Whisk the flax egg mixture before adding to the bowl with the cracker mixture. Mash using a fork until combined and the mixture is moist and crumbly. Use your hand and form the mixture into a compact ball. Transfer to a baking tray lined with parchment paper. Put another sheet of parchment paper on top. Use a

rolling pin to flatten it out with a 1/4-inch thickness. Slice into small squares using a knife or a pizza cutter. Discard the crumbs and sprinkle with sea salt all over.

3. Bake in a preheated oven at 350 degrees for 12 minutes. Flip all the pieces and bake for a minute or two.

Garlic Crackers with Thyme

Yield: 60 small crackers

Ingredients:

- 1 flax egg (combination of 3 tablespoons filtered water and 1 tablespoon ground flax)
- 1/2 teaspoon Himalayan pink salt
- 1/2 teaspoon ground black pepper
- 1/2 teaspoon ground garlic powder
- 1 tablespoon avocado oil (100 percent pure)
- 1 tablespoon freshly chopped thyme
- 2 cups almond flour

Directions:

1. Put all ingredients for the crackers in a bowl. Mix until combined.
2. Whisk the flax egg before adding to the cracker mixture. Mix well. Mash the mixture using a fork until moist and crumbly. Use your hands to shape the mixture into a compact ball. Place it on a tray lined with parchment paper. Put another sheet of parchment paper on top and roll using a rolling pin into 1/4-inch thickness. Cut into small squares using a knife or a pizza cutter.

3. Remove the crumbs and bake in a preheated oven at 350 degrees for 12 minutes. Toss the crackers and bake for 2 more minutes.

Avocado Fries

Yield: 2 to 4 servings

Ingredients:

- 1/2 cup homemade almond milk
- 2 firm avocados

For the breadcrumbs

- 1/2 teaspoon Himalayan pink salt
- 1/2 teaspoon ground smoked paprika
- 1/2 teaspoon ground garlic powder
- 1/2 cup nutritional yeast
- 1/2 cup almond flour
- 1/2 teaspoon ground cayenne pepper (optional if you want the breadcrumbs to be spicy)

Directions:

1. Put all ingredients for the breadcrumbs in a bowl. Mix until combined.
2. Slice the avocados, scoop out the meat from the skin, and slice into strips.
3. Put breadcrumbs in a bowl and non-dairy milk in another bowl. Dip the avocado strips in the bowl of milk and coat with the breadcrumb mixture.

4. Arrange the coated avocado strips in a tray lined with parchment paper. Bake in a preheated oven at 420 degrees for 10 minutes. Toss the fries and continue baking for 5 minutes or until golden brown.

5. Serve immediately.

Tasty Apple Chips

Yield: Up to 60 chips

Ingredients:

- 4 small apples (rinse and thinly slice)
- For the cinnamon mixture
- 1 teaspoon ground cinnamon
- 1 tablespoon vanilla bean powder
- 1/4 cup Xylitol (non-GMO)

Directions:

1. Put all ingredients for the cinnamon mixture in a bowl. Mix until combined.
2. Dehydrate the apple chips. Sprinkle cinnamon to both sides of an apple slice you're holding. Put in on the mesh tray of a dehydrator. Repeat the sequence until you're done with all the apple slices. Dehydrate for around 18 hours at 115 degrees.
3. Store chips in an airtight container.

Chapter 6 – Beverage and Dessert Recipes

Mint and Berry Spa Water

Yield: 1 serving

Ingredients:

- 2 fresh mint leaves
- 1/4 cup raspberries
- 1/4 cup blackberries
- 1/4 cup blueberries
- 12 ounces filtered water

Directions:

1. Put all ingredients in a glass container, cover and refrigerate overnight.

Apple and Carrot Juice

Yield: 1 serving

Ingredients:

- 1/2 lemon
- 2 stalks celery
- 1 apple
- 4 carrots

Directions:

1. Rinse and chop the vegetables. Process them in a juicer according to package instructions. Transfer to a glass. Squeeze lemon juice and stir until combined.

Celery Juice with Beet

Yield: 1 serving

Ingredients:

- 1/2 lemon
- 7 celery stalks
- 1 beet

Directions:

1. Put all ingredients in a juicer and process according to package instructions. Transfer to a glass and serve.

Hemp Protein Smoothie with Banana

Yield: 1 serving

Ingredients:

- 3 tablespoons hemp protein powder
- 1 banana
- 1 teaspoon maca powder
- 1 tablespoon spirulina powder
- 1 1/2 cups homemade almond milk

Directions:

1. Put all ingredients in a blender. Process until combined and smooth. Transfer to a glass and serve.

Vanilla Cake in a Mug

Yield: 1 serving

Ingredients:

- 1 large pastured egg (beaten)
- 1 pinch sea salt
- 1/2 teaspoon vanilla
- 1/2 teaspoon baking powder
- 1 tablespoon dark chocolate chips or seasonal fruit (optional)
- 2 teaspoons granular monk fruit sweetener
- 1 tablespoon tigernut flour
- 1 tablespoon coconut flour
- 2 tablespoons extra virgin olive oil

Directions:

1. Put tigernut flour, coconut flour, salt, baking powder, sweetener, vanilla, and oil in a heatproof mug. Mix until combined. Add egg and mix until smooth. Scrape the bottom and sides of the mug as needed. Fold in chocolate chips or chopped fruit. Microwave for a minute and 30 seconds.

2. Leave to cool, unmold, and transfer to a plate. Top with butter and serve.

Almond Balls with Cacao

Yield: 14 balls

Ingredients:

- 1/4 cup raw cacao powder
- 1/2 teaspoon vanilla bean powder
- 1 tablespoon organic date nectar
- 2 tablespoons maca powder
- 2 tablespoons hemp oil
- 1/4 cup almond flour
- 1/2 cup almond butter
- 1 cup raw almonds

Directions:

1. Put all ingredients in a food processor. Process until the consistency becomes similar to a thick paste. Adjust sweetness according to taste.

2. Spoon a mixture into your palm, roll, and shape into a ball. Repeat the process until you're done with the remaining batter. Arrange the balls on a tray. Refrigerate for at least 30 minutes before serving.

Delish Apple Pie Tart

Yield: 4 pie tarts

Ingredients:

For the crust

- 2 pinches Himalayan pink salt
- 1 teaspoon vanilla bean powder
- 4 tablespoons coconut oil
- 1 cup Medjool dates (pitted)
- 1 cup walnuts

For the filling

- 1 pinch Himalayan pink salt
- 1/8 teaspoon vanilla bean powder
- 1/4 teaspoon ground cinnamon
- 1 teaspoon lemon juice
- 2 teaspoons coconut oil
- 1 cup Medjool dates (pitted)
- 4 small red apples

Directions:

1. Put all ingredients for the crust in a food processor. Process until crumbly and sticky. Divide mixture into

4 tart dishes. Use your fingers to press the crust to the sides and bottom parts of the tart dishes.

2. Put all ingredients for the filling in a food processor. Pulse until diced. Spoon filling into each tart dish. Refrigerate for at least 30 minutes before serving.

Strawberry Shortcake

Yield: 8 servings

Ingredients:

For the topping

- 1 quart fresh strawberries (hulled and chopped)
- 1/2 teaspoon vanilla extract
- 1 tablespoon raw honey
- 1 cup grass-fed heavy cream

For the cake

- 3/4 teaspoon baking soda
- 1/2 teaspoon fine sea salt
- 3 tablespoons arrowroot starch
- 3 large pastured eggs
- 1/4 cup golden monk fruit sweetener
- 8 tablespoons unsalted butter (softened)
- 1/3 cup tigernut flour
- 1/3 cup coconut flour
- 1/2 teaspoon vanilla extract
- 1/2 lemon (grated zest)
- 1/2 cup coconut cream (whisked)

Directions:

1. Put butter and sweetener in a bowl. Mix using an electric mixer on a high-speed setting until fluffy. Turn the speed to medium and mix as you add eggs one at a time. Add vanilla, lemon zest, and coconut cream. Scrape the sides of the bowl as needed.

2. In another bowl, sift to combine the baking soda, sea salt, arrowroot starch, tigernut flour, and coconut flour. Gradually add this to the butter and egg mixture as you continue on mixing on a low-speed setting. Mix until smooth.

3. Transfer batter to a greased cake pan. Use a spatula to smoothen the top. Gently tap the pan on the counter to remove excess air. Bake in a preheated oven at 350 degrees for 35 minutes.

4. Leave on a wire rack to cool for half an hour.

5. Put cream, vanilla, and honey in a bowl. Mix using an electric mixer on a high-speed setting. Mix until soft peaks form.

6. Unmold the cake and transfer to a plate. Add the icing and spread all over. Top with sliced strawberries. Slice and serve.

Choco-Creamy Pudding

Yield: 3 cups

Ingredients:

- 1/2 cup organic date nectar
- 1 13.5-ounce can organic full-fat coconut milk
- 1 teaspoon vanilla bean powder
- 1/4 cup raw cacao powder
- 4 avocados (pitted)

Directions:

1. Refrigerate the can of coconut milk the night before you prepare the recipe.
2. Scoop out the coconut fat from the can and reserve the liquid for another recipe. Transfer the coconut fat to a blender. Add the rest of the ingredients and process until smooth.
3. Transfer to a bowl and serve at once.

Pecan Pie Bites

Yield: 8 small bites

Ingredients:

- 1/2 teaspoon vanilla bean powder
- 8 Medjool dates (pitted)
- 1 cup pecans

Directions:

1. Put all ingredients in a food processor. Process until sticky and crumbly.
2. Spoon a mixture into your palm. Squeeze to make it compact and roll into a ball. Repeat the sequence until you're done with the rest of the mixture.
3. Arrange balls on a plate. Refrigerate for at least 15 minutes before serving.

Strawberry Mousse

Yield: 1 to 2 servings

Ingredients:

- 2 tablespoons Xylitol (non-GMO)
- 3 tablespoons freeze-dried strawberries
- 1 13.5-ounce can organic full-fat coconut milk

Directions:

1. Refrigerate the can of coconut milk overnight. Scoop out the hardened fat and put in a bowl. Reserve the liquid part for a smoothie recipe.
2. Add freeze-dried strawberries and Xylitol to the coconut fat. Mix on a high speed until thick and fluffy.
3. Serve at once.

Conclusion

Thank you again for downloading this book!

I hope this book was able to help you to prepare the right meals suited for a lectin-free diet. This diet, aside from weight loss, also helps those who are suffering from metabolic syndrome and cardiovascular disease.

Like any kinds of diet, the idea here is to eat in moderation. It is also best to team up the diet with exercise and healthy lifestyle to speed up the weight loss process and make it easier for you to maintain your ideal figure.

Printed in Great Britain
by Amazon